Insulin Resistance Diet

The Ultimate Beginners Guide To Overcome Insulin Resistance, Control Blood Sugar Levels, and Lose Weight to Live a Healthier and more Vibrant Life

Table of Contents

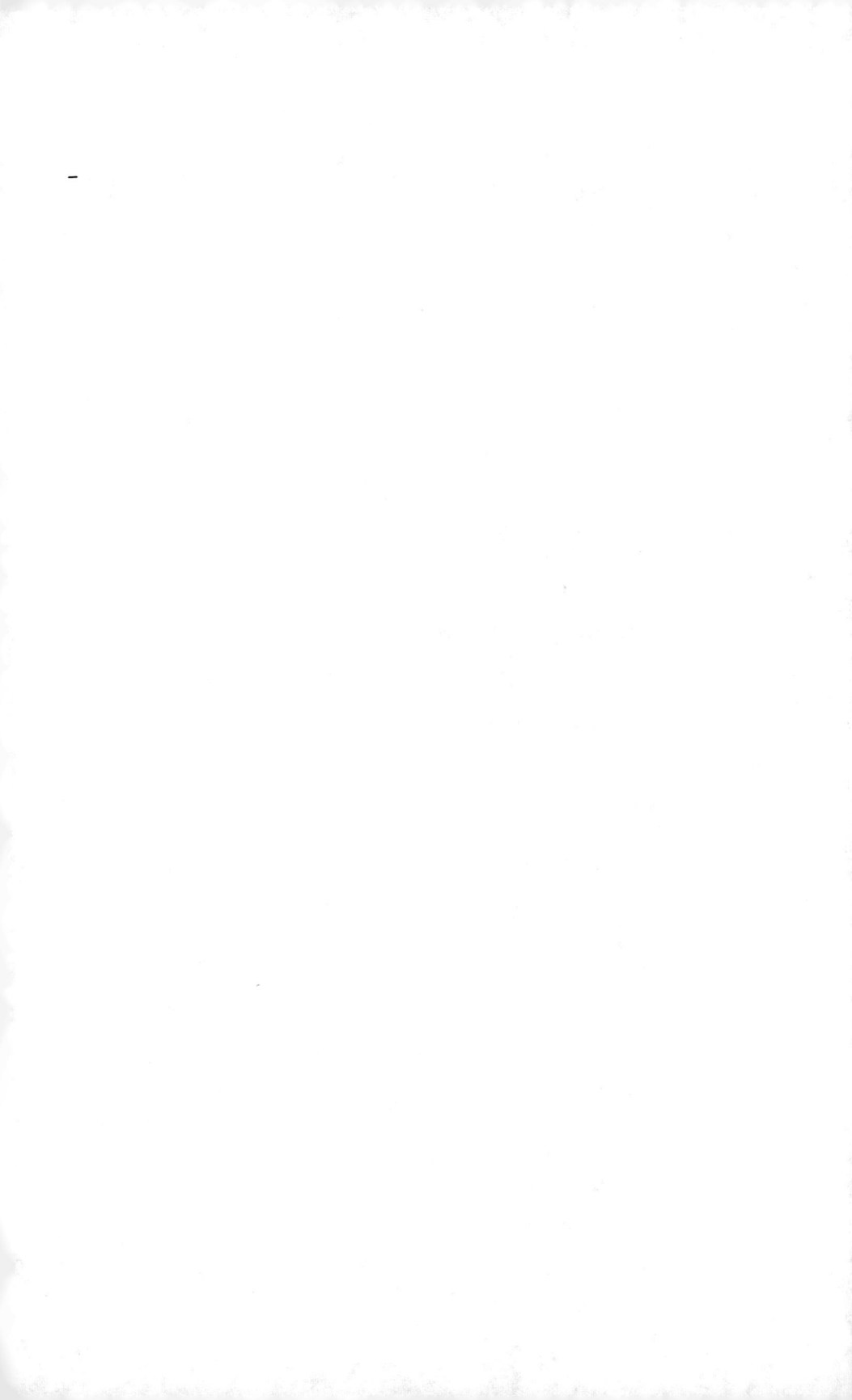

Introduction

Having insulin resistance can be quite scary,
but fortunately, it doesn't necessarily have to
leave a significant effect on your overall health.
Sure, it is a fact that insulin resistance can lead
to type 2 diabetes, but who says that that has to
happen? If you left your doctor's office
frightened by the news that you are affected by
this condition, well, let me cheer you up and
tell you that there is absolutely no need to
worry.

If you think that the tragic news you have just
received mean that from now on you are
sentenced to eat tasteless food and be deprived
of the enjoyment of eating delightful delicacies
in order to maintain your health, then you
cannot be more wrong. And to convince you in
what I just said, I present to you this guide. The
only guide that will allow you to munch on
deliciousness burn fat, lose weight and most

importantly, keep your blood sugar in check, all at the same time. This is not a diet guide with tons of restrictions. This is a guide that offers endless possibilities.

From what role does insulin resistance plays, to why it is important to start a Ketogenic diet with some finger-licking recipes for one week's meal plan, this book will help you reverse your insulin resistance.
Now go on, read and see why it is definitely the ultimate guide.

This document is geared towards providing exact and reliable information in regards to the topic and issue covered. The publication is sold with the idea that the publisher is not required to render accounting, officially permitted, or otherwise, qualified services. If advice is necessary, legal or professional, a practiced individual in the profession should be ordered.

- From a Declaration of Principles which was accepted and approved equally by a Committee of the American Bar Association and a Committee of Publishers and Associations.

The information provided herein is stated to be truthful and consistent, in that any liability, in terms of inattention or otherwise, by any usage or abuse of any policies, processes, or directions contained within is the solitary and utter responsibility of the recipient reader. Under no circumstances will any legal responsibility or blame be held against the publisher for any reparation, damages, or monetary loss due to the information herein, either directly or indirectly.

Respective authors own all copyrights not held by the publisher.

The information herein is offered for informational purposes solely, and is universal as so. The presentation of the information is without contract or any type of guarantee assurance.

The trademarks that are used are without any consent, and the publication of the trademark is without permission or backing by the trademark owner. All trademarks and brands within this book are for clarifying purposes only and are the owned by the owners themselves, not affiliated with this document.

Explaining Insulin Resistance

Who doesn't want to eat? I really don't know a single person who doesn't enjoy a delicious Italian pasta. Top it with mozzarella and Parmesan cheese and I can see the bottom of the bowl before you count to 3. We all love the explosion of flavors that happens on our tongues when we start chewing those 'little' bites. Hey, that's the whole point of offering a ton of different pasta choices on the menu. We all crave the delightful taste. Okay, so, we have a nice dinner and the next thing we know, our gut stops rambling. But what happens inside our tummies after we swallow that pasta dish? Here is what happen when we eat carbohydrates. As we all know carbohydrates are all types of sugar (honey included), fruits and starchy food, yes, in this case, that bowl of spaghetti. Once we ingest the delicious pasta meal, the body starts to slowly digest it. During digestion, the carbohydrates are being broken down into sugars, and as we all know, the simplest one of all is glucose. So, normally, after such a carb-loaded meal, the blood glucose levels increase.

So what is the insulin's role in all of this? Insulin is a hormone that is made in the pancreas that has a major part in our metabolism. It allows our muscles, fat, and liver to absorb the glucose levels from the blood. It also helps the muscle and liver to store the excess sugar from the blood, and it decreases the liver's production of glucose. So, in short, without insulin, our blood sugar levels would be sky-scraping.

Got the picture? Now, let's explain what happens when someone has insulin resistance. Insulin resistance is a condition when the liver, fat, and muscle simply cannot respond to insulin the way they should, meaning that the blood sugar cannot be that easily absorbed. As a result of this improper reaction of the muscle, liver, and fat to insulin, the body needs an increased amount of insulin in order to keep the blood glucose levels in check. So the body sends signals to the pancreas to increase its production of insulin, and the beta cells try to keep up with the high demand so it produces more of the hormone, so that the cells will stay energized and the blood sugar under control.

Before I go any further, I would like to clear something up as I have found out that many people have uncertainties regarding this condition. Insulin resistance is not the same as diabetes. It is simply a condition where the body needs an increased amount of insulin to keep the glucose in the bloodstream in check. So where is the problem? The problem with insulin resistance is that this elevated production of the insulin can eventually lead to wearing off the beta cells in charge of producing this hormone and the resistance will get worse. The insufficient amount of insulin means improper glucose absorption, which means elevated glucose levels in the bloodstream (prediabetes), which will eventually lead to type 2 diabetes. However, the association of insulin resistance with diabetes and other conditions that it is linked with, cannot be fully understood, simply because there isn't a known pattern in which this condition develops. Insulin resistance can lead to diabetes, but not always, just as some people with diabetes are insulin resistant and others are not. Fingers crossed the mystery will be solved anytime soon.

The Cause

Usually, any medical condition can be linked to a list of factors that may contribute to its occurrence. That is not the case with insulin resistance. However, to say that insulin resistance is a condition that occurs as a result of a single cause is a mistake. Insulin resistance is a health-concerning problem that experts have been struggling to decipher for many years now. After blaming every possible tissue in our body and looking for the culprit in the most obvious places like the pancreas, muscle, and liver, scientists have come to the point to accept that insulin resistance is an extremely complex metabolic disorder.

The general public, usually those affected by this condition, is really offered little information on this subject, and understandably more and more people start to think how the information is intentionally 'hidden' so that the pharmaceutical world and health organizations can profit from diseases such as diabetes. No matter how much this might make sense to you, approaching such a serious condition with a pessimistic mind frame is not the solution.

Although no one can pinpoint the exact reason for insulin resistance, health experts agree that the fat we eat pulls the strings and can cause this condition. A high-fat diet, excess weight and the inability to 'burn' fat, are mainly responsible for this vexing condition.

The Extra Pounds – Experts used to believe how the fat tissue was nothing more but a place where our body stored energy, but after years of research and many clinical studies, it is now known that the fat around the belly is primarily guilty for causing many conditions, since it produces some substances and hormones that can cause insulin resistance, high cholesterol, high blood pressure, etc.

Obesity is believed to be one of the main reasons why this condition may occur. Central obesity (around the belly) is primarily guilty for depriving the fat cells of oxygen and forcing them to die, which makes the body react with an inflammatory response, which of course contributes to insulin resistance.

Being Inactive – Since extra fat can be the cause, it is only understandable how being physically inactive can also contribute to insulin resistance. Muscle uses more blood sugar than any other tissues in our body. If we keep the muscles active, they will do their job properly and burn the stored glucose, making room for new blood sugar, which will keep the blood glucose levels in check. Many studies have also shown that after physical activity, our muscles become super sensitive to insulin, which can only reverse a condition like insulin resistance.

Are You Affected?

The tricky part about having insulin resistance is the fact that it is a silent condition. It doesn't trigger any symptoms that may cause worry or concern in the beginning. What do I mean in the beginning? I mean in the early phases before it advances to prediabetes. There isn't a possible way to detect insulin resistance on your own, simply because it shows no clear signs, unlike diabetes when there is a list of symptoms that may convince you to do a medical checkup.

However, even though there aren't any signs that may indicate the existence of insulin resistance, doing some tests and checking your insulin sensitivity cannot hurt you. You should especially be concerned about the possible occurrence of this condition if:

- You are overweight (especially around the abdomen)

- You are older than 40

- You have high cholesterol

- You have high blood pressure

- You have PCOS (Polycystic Ovary Syndrome)

- You live a sedentary lifestyle

- You have a family history of diabetes

- You had a baby who was heavier than 9 pounds

Although in the early stages, there aren't any indications of insulin resistance, once it advances, this condition can result in:

- High blood sugar

- Fatty liver

- High blood pressure

- Acne and large face pores

- Extreme hunger and food cravings

- Swollen ankles

- Apple-shaped figure

- Skin tags

- Hair loss

Insulin resistance never happens overnight. There isn't a single thing you can do that will trigger the insulin levels to suddenly rise to that point that you will become insulin resistant. This condition happens slowly, gradually and over time. Once a person becomes affected, he/she cannot know it, unless he/she gets tested. So why don't we all? Now, that is the question of the century. Why don't doctors express concerns about this condition? Why don't they suggest these kinds of tests to the patients? Whether it is for purely economic reasons, or simply because they have been trained that way is up for a debate, and a subject for a different time and place. Be as it may, one thing is for sure. Once the blood sugar levels skyrocket, it is a little too late. Why wait for the numbers of the monitor to scare us to death? Don't wait for you to show symptoms of diabetes so that your doctor suggests a fasting blood sugar test. From time to time, checking yourself for insulin resistance will not do you any harm. In some cases, that one decision can be life-saving.

The glucose tolerance test is the most reliable test for insulin resistance. It is a test when the patient is given glucose and when blood samples are taken in order to detect the way in which the glucose is absorbed. This will indicate whether the insulin does its job properly or not. Usually, this test is done within 2 hours. First the blood glucose is checked while the patient is fasting, and then again at 1 and 2 hour intervals.

Measuring the lipid hormones can also give a pretty good insight of the fat metabolism and insulin relationship.

If your test results show insulin resistance, it doesn't mean that you are in danger, but that you have dodged a bullet, since knowing this condition before it advances into something

more dangerous gives you a pretty good lead
and the chance to do the right thing to reverse
it.

Reversing It Naturally

After explaining this condition, I think everyone got the point and learned that the only possible way to reverse insulin resistance is through a healthy diet and balanced lifestyle. Since the insulin is in charge of persuading muscle, liver, and fat to absorb the glucose, and when there is insulin resistance they are kind of disobeying this hormone, limiting the sugar intake is more than crucial in order to stop it from piling up in the blood and result in diabetes.

Needless to say, but the solution is simple. That chocolate icing cake may put a smile on your face, but it will also kill the fat cells in your belly and will create a pouch, which let's face it, despite the fact that it will not look good in that new shirt you bought the other day, it will also increase the insulin spikes and contribute to more serious health complications.

And is there a better way to approach such a condition than with what nature has to offer? In my opinion, the natural approach is the only weapon you will ever need when fighting a war like this. People in the past didn't know of another way to treat a condition. Why do we always try to take the 'easy way out'? Why do we think that popping pills will solve our problems? Read on to find out how to reverse insulin resistance naturally.

Beware the Culprits

The truth is, whenever your cells are exposed to insulin, they become more insulin resistant. That is an inevitable fact, and there is absolutely nothing you can do to change the course in which the process of absorbing the glucose from the bloodstream works. However, we can indeed do a lot that can help us. We can reverse insulin resistance and improve our overall health by paying attention to the food we ingest. By making sure that the pancreas will not get such an increased demand for producing insulin, we can move towards a much healthier life.

But where do we start? How to know what shouldn't be put on our dinner tables? What food requires an increased release of insulin? Here is what should be tossed in your garbage can immediately if you want to stop this condition for messing with your general health:

Sugar. Is it really necessary for me to explain this? It is clear as day that people with insulin resistance should purge this sweet hazard from their diets. When I say purge, I mean say goodbye to sugar for good. And no, honey is not the healthier choice, not for you anyway.

Trans Fats. If you are looking for the unhealthiest type of fats, let me introduce you to trans fats. When hydrogen is added to unsaturated fats, trans fats are born. Besides that they cause inflammation, next to sugar, they are the second enemy to your insulin sensitivity. You will mostly find this kind of fats in cans and packages.

Bad Carbs. Since there is an ongoing debate and misunderstanding regarding which type of carbs are good and which are bad, let me explain the confusion. Some may think how potatoes are bad since they are carb-loaded, well this is not entirely true. You see, a single potato weighing 6 ounces it is mostly made of water; only 23% of its entire weight are carbs. On the other hand, a rice cake may weigh 1/5 ounce, but 80% of its weight is carbohydrate. The bad carbs are mostly found in bread, bagels, white rice, pasta, crackers, cereals, etc.

High-Lactose Dairy. Some may disagree with this, but it is the truth. Milk and other high-dairy products torment our tummies, making the pounds stick around our abdomen and contribute to insulin resistance. How? As any other type of food, when we ingest lactose, it is broken down by the lactase enzyme. So where is the problem? The problem is that as we grow older, our body produces less of the lactase enzyme, and it makes it hard for our bodies to digest lactose.

Gluten. Grains, such as wheat, are made of a sticky protein called gluten that is surely unfriendly, not only to your body shape but also to your health, since it is known that it can elevate the blood sugar, which you want to avoid at all costs. Gluten also leads to inflammation, which is yet another reason to keep it off your kitchen.

Soda. If you thought that you could trick your gut by satisfying your sweet tooth and drinking a fizzy drink, you were wrong. Besides the obvious fact of keeping your blood sugar in check, you should also avoid soda because it has a huge contribution to gaining weight. And in case you were wondering, no, switching to diet coke is not a healthy alternative.

Processed Meat. Processed meat may bring out some amazing flavors to your sandwich, but it is not kind to your health. It is packed with calories that will wrap your belly and contribute to insulin resistance. Besides that, it contains additives and nitrates that may cause additional health problems.

Beware the Organic Trap. These days, you can buy just about anything in 'organic' version. But just because the label says it's organic it doesn't mean that it is healthy for you. By eating organic cookies, you are adding to your belly weight and supporting insulin resistance, the same way as if you were eating regular chocolate cookies.

Your Kitchen Must Haves

Just like there is a list of food that should be off limits for those trying to reverse insulin resistance and get their tissues to absorb the blood glucose the way they should, there is also a long list of foods that should be a part of their kitchen and pantry. I am talking about the healthy choices. The food that contributes to lowering blood sugar and improving the insulin sensitivity.

Having insulin resistance doesn't mean that there will be nothing but green vegetables in your fridge. In fact, you will be surprised to know about the variety of delicious foods that should be a part of your diet. Thinking that you will not enjoy cooking again? Well, think again, because you better throw these food items in the shopping cart the next time you visit the supermarket.

Omega 3 Fatty Acids. Although it is long believed that omega 3 fatty acids have the potential to somehow improve the insulin sensitivity, now it is known how. Omega 3 fatty acids interact with the cell receptors in a way that they allow them to bind more of the hormone insulin easily and therefore help reverse insulin resistance. You can find omega 3 fatty acids in cold water fish like salmon, sardines, trout, tuna, herring, oyster. This is excellent news for the fish lovers, but for those of you who don't eat fish, make sure to substitute it with some omega 3fatty acid supplement, since theses acids play a major role in reversing insulin resistance.

Fruits and Vegetables. Now, we all know the importance of fresh fruit and vegetables in our diet, whether we are suffering from a health condition or not. However, those who want to control and reverse their insulin resistance should make sure to follow this diet rule, since most of the studies regarding this and similar conditions have shown that eating a variety of fruits and veggies help in improving the overall health. Here is what you absolutely must have in your kitchen:

Blueberries – Thanks to their chemical called anthocyanins, blueberries stimulate the release of adiponectin, which helps the body to increase its sensitivity to insulin and lower the blood glucose.

Leafy Green Vegetables – Spinach, broccoli, kale, collard greens and other leafy greens play a major role in reversing insulin resistance and repairing damaged blood vessels. They are amazing antioxidants, rich in fiber and real vitamin bombs.

Indian Gooseberry – Also called amla fruit, Indian gooseberry is one of the most important natural cure in the Ayurvedic medicine. It promotes a proper pancreas function and boosts insulin sensitivity.

Always aim for fruits and veggies with a low glycemic index such as avocado, tomatoes, berries, onions, citrus fruit, mushrooms, grapes, nectarines, asparagus, etc.

If you cannot find some types of fruit or vegetables to buy fresh, know that the frozen option is just as healthy.

Whole Grains. According to many studies (most of them published in the European Journal of Clinical Nutrition), implementing whole grains into your diet can contribute to reversing insulin resistance, or reducing the risk for those not affected by this condition. Barley, whole wheat, oats, bulgur, and spelt, support the managing of the blood sugar and improving the insulin sensitivity. So, throw that cereal package away and enjoy a healthy oatmeal for breakfast instead.

Nuts. Nuts, especially walnuts, should be an important part of your path to reversing insulin resistance. According to a study performed by the University of California, walnuts boost insulin sensitivity, contribute to managing the blood sugar levels, lower cholesterol and can slow down the growth of a prostate cancer.

Legumes. Legumes are known to have the power to manage the levels of glucose in the blood, but not only diabetics can benefit from adding them to their meals. People who are insulin resistant should also make lentils, peas, chickpeas and beans, especially cannelloni beans, a significant part of their diet since they can make the muscle, liver, and fat respond to insulin more effectively.

Monounsaturated Fats. Monounsaturated fats are those kinds of fats that are found in the plants. They can be found in olive oil, canola oil, walnut oil, avocados, nuts, and seeds, etc. Nut butters are a great choice for insulin resistant people since they are monounsaturated, contribute to controlling the insulin sensitivity and can provide you with enough proteins to keep your tummy full and energize you.

Spices. If you enjoy spicing up your meals, then here are some good news for you – go ahead. There are many spices that can contribute to reversing insulin resistance.

Cinnamon – This flavorful spice increases our ability to respond to insulin, and therefore must be a part of an insulin resistance diet. There are many heavy clinical studies that have shown how cinnamon reduces the fasting blood sugar levels. If you implement less than a half a teaspoon of cinnamon each day, it will have a significant impact on your improving insulin goal.

Turmeric – The curcumin compound found in turmeric is a powerful antioxidant packed with anti-inflammatory properties. A study published in Molecular Nutrition & Food Research says that turmeric has an important effect in preventing problems associated with insulin resistance such as liver diseases.

Ginger, fenugreek, garlic, cayenne pepper, cumin, and ginseng are other spices that are known to help manage the blood sugar and control insulin resistance.

Herbs and Leaves. There are many herbs, leaves and leave extracts that can contribute to improving your health by managing the insulin and blood sugar levels.

Mango Leaves – Used for centuries as a remedy in Chinese medicine, mango leaves are a great addition to your diet, since they can help you regulate the insulin and control the blood glucose levels. And implementing mango leaves in your diet couldn't be simpler; just boil 2-3 leaves in a cup of water, drink the tea warm, and enjoy.

Spirulina – Although not so much an herb, actually an acyanobacteria, spirulina is a blueish green algae that is safe to consume. You can find it in a powder form in most well-equipped health stores. Research shows that spirulina can improve insulin sensitivity by an incredible 225%.

Green Tea. Many studies have shown that the antioxidant called epigallocatechin gallate that can be found in green tea can promote proper insulin activity and keep the blood sugar levels in check. Thinking about a cup of tea? Make it green.

Olive Leaf Extract. A research performed by the University of Aukland has found that the extract from the olive leaves can nudge the pancreas to increase its production of insulin, which can clearly contribute to controlling and eventually reversing the insulin resistance.

Natural Supplements

If you are against drugs (and you should be, unless of course, your condition requires some serious treatment) you can talk to your physician about the alternative of adding natural supplements to your diet.

Magnesium. People that are insulin resistant are usually deprived of this essential nutrient. Magnesium is known to regulate the insulin sensitivity and contribute to managing the blood sugar.

Vanadium. If you are looking for a mineral that will surely optimize the glucose tolerance, then that's vanadium. Vanadium works in an almost exact way as the insulin, and that is why it is said that it mimics it. Studies have shown that vanadium can increase the insulin sensitivity and decrease the body fat and the appetite at the same time.

Chromium. One of the essential minerals that can enhance the activity of the insulin and lower the risk of cardiovascular diseases. Although it is normal for our cells to be more deficient of this mineral as we grow old, it is proven that people with insulin resistance and type 2 diabetes have significantly lower chromium levels than those who are not affected by these conditions. Talk to your doctor and see if there is a need for you to take a chromium supplement.

Berberine. Berberine is a compound that can be found in the roots of some plants such as Oregon grape, barberry, and goldenseal. Its association with insulin resistance is simple. Berberine can lower the blood sugar and decrease the demand for insulin production, which can improve insulin sensitivity. People suffering from diabetes are encouraged to take berberine supplement since there are many studies that have found that this beneficial compound can actually be as effective as diabetes drugs, without the possible side effects, of course.

Garcinia Cambogia. Although it is primarily a weight-loss aid since it decreases the hunger, diabetics and people who are insulin resistant can indeed benefit from supplementing their diet with Garcinia Cambogia. The hydroxycitric acid that Garcinia Cambogia contains can delay the absorption of the blood glucose levels after meals, which can clearly improve the glucose metabolism. This acid orders the liver to store more glucose levels than the fat.

Never take supplements on your own, even if they are natural. Be especially careful if you are already taking medications since it is known that supplements can interfere with some medicaments. Express your wish to your doctor, and ask him/her to prescribe the best possible supplement for your condition.

Go 'Keto'

Ketogenic diet. More and more health gurus are recommending it and nowadays, this diet is one of the most common worldwide. If you go to a bookstore and quickly skim through the pages of a couple of cookbooks, chances are, the word 'keto' will pop up sooner rather than later. Okay, we can all agree that even if not all of us are aware of what a person on a 'keto' diet eats, we have all heard about this diet. So, what does a keto meal include? And what does ketogenic diet have to do with insulin resistance?

A ketogenic diet is a diet that consists of food that is high in fat and low in carbohydrates. You must be confused now since I have been talking about how important getting rid of the fat is from chapter 1, but let me explain this to you. With the ketogenic diet, you will be doing both, eating and losing the fat, while obviously, reversing your insulin resistance. Now you must wonder how that's possible. You see, if you choose to be on a ketogenic diet, you will switch the carb-loaded foods you usually consume with high-fat foods with moderate protein. The whole point is to minimize the carbohydrate intake as much as we can, but at the same time, receive all of the important nutrients and stay energized. But, won't the fat stick to our bellies and thighs, and increase our weight? The answer is – no. On the contrary, with the ketogenic diet, you will also shed some pounds. Okay, but won't the high-fat diet boost our glucose levels? Again, the answer is – definitely no. And here is why. Fats have really a non-significant impact on our insulin activity and blood sugar levels. High-protein foods, on the other hand, can easily spike the insulin levels and raise the blood sugar.

When the intake of carbohydrates is pretty small, the body is forced to burn fats a lot faster than carbs. As we said in the beginning, normally, the carbs are converted into glucose, which is then transferred through the bloodstream. But, when there is such a limited intake of carbs, the liver converts the fat into fatty acids and then ketones. These ketone bodies are transferred to the brain to work as an energy source and replace the glucose.

The ketogenic diet was created in 1924 by Dr. Russel Wilder at the Mayo Clinic, and its primary goal was to treat epilepsy. The most amazing thing about it is that other than the fact that it forbids carb-loaded food, it has no special restrictions. You don't have to go venturing down the healthy-and-organic aisle in the supermarket and buy some special low-carb food. The only trick? Ketogenic diet requires whole and unprocessed foods, so if you have absolutely no idea how to cook, this is probably the time to purchase a cooking-for-beginners kind of book and work on your cooking skills, if you want to decrease the fat distribution and improve your insulin sensitivity.

There are many studies that have shown how the ketogenic diet is beneficial for the people suffering from insulin resistance, but most of these researches were mainly performed on middle-aged and obese subjects. In 2014 a study was performed on 8 male subjects who were young, with average weight and were athletes. The ketogenic diet was compared with an experimental diet that consisted of 50% of carbs, 30% of fat and 20% of protein. The researchers found that a low-carb diet, in this case ketogenic, can improve the insulin activity, can reduce the body mass, reduces the fat content, plus it also improves athletic performance.

There are many other studies who have shown that the low-carb diets are really superior to the low-fat meal plans when it comes to enhancing the insulin sensitivity.

The ketogenic diet has a nutrient intake of:

70 % of fat

20 % of the calories are from protein

10 % of carbohydrate

*Know that the fat intake isn't the bad type such as trans fats. Ketogenic diet requires beneficial fats, such as coconut oil, avocado, grass-pastured butter, raw nuts, etc.

*Ketogenic diet also consists of dietary products, but since we said how high-fat dairy should be avoided as it can contribute to weight-gaining, be careful of what type of the dairy products you will be using.

Clean Your Diet

Have you emptied your fridge yet? The first step towards a clean diet that will help you reverse your insulin resistance is, of course, cleaning your kitchen. That means, fridge, pantry, everything. Yes, even that top shelf where the sweet and hazardous satisfactions hide. That one especially. Having these 'distractions' lying around your kitchen you can easily reach out for comfort when in a low mood, and the last thing you would possibly want is for those carb-loaded muffins to knock down multiple days of dieting.

7-Day Meal Plan

After cleaning your kitchen, you can easily clean your diet. Having bought all of the previously mentioned must haves, and being supplied with vitamins, minerals and all of the necessary nutrients, you can now safely embark the journey of reversing insulin resistance. But where to start? What to eat now? Being separated from the things you used to cook, it is understandable how full, but at the same time so empty your fridge may look to you at this point. But, don't worry because this guide will provide you with an amazing way to start. Below you will find a meal plan for a whole week, that will help you understand what and how to cook on an insulin resistance diet. Make these delicious recipes, and let them also serve you as a motivation that will trigger your creativity and inspire to come up with your own delightful meals.

Breakfast Recipes

You know what they say - breakfast is the most important meal of the day. As such, it should energize you and help you start your day the right way. Being on an insulin resistance diet doesn't mean that you get to starve. Here are 7 amazing recipes that will show you that your new diet can be just as delicious.

Day 1: Pumpkin Pancakes

Ingredients:

2 ounces of ground Hazelnuts

2 ounces of ground Flax Seeds

1 ounce Egg White Protein

3 Organic Eggs

1 tbsp Chai Masala Mix

½ cup Pumpkin Puree

1 tsp Vanilla Extract

1 tsp aluminum free Baking Powder

Slices of Fresh Fruit

Coconut Oil for frying

· Preparation:

1. Place all of the wet ingredients in a bowl and mix for about 30 seconds.

2. In another bowl, combine the masala mix, hazelnuts, flax seeds and baking powder.

3. While whisking, gradually add the wet ingredients to the dry.

4. The batter should be semi-thick. Add a little bit of water if needed.

5. Heat 1 tsp of coconut oil in a nonstick pan over medium heat.

6. Add approximately a ladle to the pan.

7. Cook the pancakes for about 2-3 minutes on each side.

8. Top with slices of fresh fruit.

9. Enjoy.

Day 2: Fishermen's Eggs

Ingredients:

2 Organic Eggs

½ cup of Arugula

2 ½ tbsp marinated Artichoke Hearts

2 ounces of Sardines in Olive Oil

Fresh Black Pepper

Preparation:

1. Preheat your oven to 375 degrees F.

2. Place the sardines in the bottom of two heatproof stonewares.

3. Break the eggs over the sardines.

4. Place the arugula over the eggs.

5. Top with artichokes.

6. Sprinkle with black pepper.

7. Bake for about 10 minutes, or as desired.

8. Enjoy.

Day 3: Red Velvet Smoothie

Ingredients:

2 cups of Coconut or Almond Milk

½ Avocado

½ small Beet

3 tbsp Cacao Powder, unsweetened

2 cups of Ice Cubes

½ tsp Vanilla Extract

A Handful of Blueberries

Preparation:

1. Place all of the ingredients in a blender.

2. Process until smooth.

3. Enjoy.

Day 4: Kale and Chives Egg Muffins

Ingredients:

6 Organic Eggs

¼ cup Chives, chopped

½ cup Coconut Milk

1 cup of Kale, finely chopped

Ground Black Pepper, to taste

Preparation:

1. Preheat your oven to 350 degrees F.

2. Whisk the eggs.

3. Stir in the chives and kale.

4. Add the coconut milk.

5. Season with black pepper, to taste.

6. Divide the mixture between 8 muffin tins.

7. Bake for about half an hour.

8. Leave the muffins to cool, before lifting them with a fork.

9. Enjoy.

Day 5: Breakfast Mix

Ingredients:

5 tbsp of Flax Seeds

7 tbsp of Hemp Seeds

5 tbsp of Coconut Flakes, unsweetened

2 tbsp of Sesame Seeds

2 tbsp dark Cocoa Powder, unsweetened

Almond Milk or Stil Water

Preparation:

1. Grind the sesame and hemp seeds for a short time, as you don't want to make a paste.

2. Place them into a jar.

3. Add all of the remaining ingredients to the jar.

4. Close the lid and shake the jar well, to combine.

5. Serve a couple of tablespoons of the mix with almond milk, or even with still water.

6. Keep the breakfast mix refrigerated, as the seeds have a high fat content.

7. Enjoy.

Day 6: Avocado and Salmon Boats

Ingredients:

1 Ripe Avocado (about 2 ½ ounces)

1 ounce of Fresh and Organic Goat Cheese

2 ounces of Smoked Salmon (wild caught)

2 tbsp of Extra Virgin Olive Oil

Juice of 1 Lemon

Ground Black Pepper, to taste

Preparation:

1. Halve the avocado and remove its seed.

2. Place all of the remaining ingredients in a food processor.

3. Process until they are coarsely chopped.

4. Place the mixture in the avocado halves.

5. Sprinkle with black pepper.

You can also:

6. Cut the avocado into cubes.

7. Slice the salmon into pieces.

8. Place them in a bowl.

9. Stir in the goat cheese.

10. Sprinkle with black pepper.

11.Enjoy.

Day 7: Mini Frittatas

Ingredients:

8 ounces ground Beef

2 cups of diced Red and Yellow Bell Peppers

½ cup Almond Milk

½ cup Pepper Jack Cheese

10 Organic Eggs plus 2 Egg Whites

¼ tsp Black Pepper

1/4 cup of finely chopped Cilantro

1 tbsp Olive Oil

Preparation:

1. Preheat your oven to 350 degrees F.

2. In a skillet, heat the olive oil over medium heat.

3. Add the meat and cook it until brown.

4. Remove the meat from the skillet; set aside.

5. In the same skillet, sauté the peppers for 3 minutes, or until soft.

6. Whisk the eggs, egg whites and almond milk in a large bowl.

7. Divide the beef and peppers between muffin tins evenly.

8. Add chopped cilantro.

9. Pour the egg mixture over.

10. Carefully stir the mixture with a fork.

11. Sprinkle with cheese.

12. Bake for about half an hour.

13. Allow to cool before you lift the frittata with a fork.

14. Enjoy.

Lunch Recipes

If you thought that your lunch would be nothing but fresh green salad from now on, well, think again. These next 7 recipes will prove you that cooking on an insulin resistance diet is surely not boring. Plus, they are so easy to pack and bring to work.

Day 1: Flourless Crab Cakes

Ingredients:

1 pound of Crab Meat

2 Green Onions, finely chopped

¼ cup chopped Fresh Cilantro

¼ cup chopped Fresh Parsley

1 tsp finely chopped seeded Jalapeno Pepper, optional

1 tsp of Lemon Juice

½ tsp of powdered Mustard

1 large Organic Egg

2 tbsp Olive Oil

A pinch of Black Pepper

Preparation:

1. Place the previously cleaned crab meat in a bowl.

2. Add onions, cilantro, parsley, jalapeno, mustard and lemon juice to the meat.

3. Stir to combine, but be careful not to break the lumps of the crab.

4. Beat the egg in a small bowl.

5. Add it to the mixture.

6. Cover the bowl with a plastic wrap and refrigerate the mixture for a couple of hours.

7. Discard the excess liquid.

8. Shape 6 crab cakes.

9. Place them on a baking sheet.

10. Heat half of the olive oil in a skillet over medium heat.

11. Place 3 crabs in the skillet and cook for about 3 minutes.

12. Turn them over and bake for additional 3 minutes.

13. Repeat with the remaining oil and crabs.

14. Enjoy.

Day 2: Fennel Walnut Chicken Salad

Ingredients:

3 cooked Chicken Breasts, diced

2 tbsp Walnut Oil

2 tbsp Fennel Fronds, chopped

¼ cup toasted Walnuts, chopped

1 ½ cup fresh Fennel, chopped

2 Garlic Cloves, pressed

1/8 tsp Cayenne Pepper

2 tbsp Lemon Juice

Preparation:

1. In a bowl, place the chicken, fennel, and walnuts.

2. Toss to combine.

3. In a smaller bowl, whisk the lemon juice, fennel fronds, garlic and cayenne pepper.

4. Pour the lemon mixture over the salad.

5. Stir until it is well-coated.

6. Refrigerate for an hour.

7. Enjoy.

Day 3: Thai Coconut Soup

Ingredients:

For the Broth:

1 ½ cups Coconut Milk

4 cups Chicken Broth

1 cup Fresh Cilantro

1 inch piece of Fresh Ginger

Zest of 1 Lime

For the Soup:

4 ounces Wild Caught Shrimp

1 Anchovy, smashed

1 tbsp Coconut Oil

1 ounce Mushrooms

1 ounce sliced Onions

Juice of 1 Lime

Preparation:

1. Place all of the broth ingredients in a saucepan.

2. Simmer for 20 minutes.

3. Strain the mixture through a fine mesh and return back to the pan.

4. Bring it back to a simmer.

5. Add the shrimp and anchovy.

6. Stir in the mushrooms and onions.

7. Simmer for 10 minutes.

8. Add the lime juice.

9. Serve and enjoy.

Day 4: Southern Coleslaw

Ingredients:

½ Cabbage Head, shredded

3 tbsp Apple Cider Vinegar

½ tsp Celery Seed

1 cup Mayonnaise

1 cup thinly sliced Celery

¼ tsp liquid Stevia

Preparation:

1. Place the celery and cabbage in a large bowl.

2. Stir in the mayonnaise, stevia, celery seed and vinegar in a small bowl.

3. Pour the dressing over the cabbage and celery.

4. Refrigerate for a couple of hours.

5. Enjoy.

Day 5: Lime Chicken Crockpot Chowder

Ingredients:

1 small Onion, diced

Juice of 1 Lime

1 pound of boneless and skinless Chicken Thighs

8 ounces Cream Cheese

1 can Diced Tomatoes

1 Garlic Clove, pressed

1 tbsp Pepper

1 cup of Chicken Broth

Preparation:

1. Place all of the ingredients in a crock pot.

2. Cook for at least 4 hours.

3. Shred the cooked chicken inside of the pot.

4. Serve and enjoy.

Day 6: Dill Tuna Sandwich

Ingredients;

Long Sliced Dills

1 can of Tuna

1 pinch of dried Dill

3 tbsp Mayonnaise

Black Pepper, to taste

Preparation:

1. Place all of the ingredients, except the dills, into a bowl.

2. Stir to combine.

3. Place some of the tuna mixture on top of one dill.

4. Top with another.

5. Place a toothpick to keep your sandwiches together.

6. Repeat until you use all of the tuna mixture.

7. Enjoy.

Day 7: Steak and Chimichurri Salad

Ingredients:

4 ounces Cooked Steak, sliced

2 Radishes, thinly sliced

1/3 cup Red cabbage, shredded

2 cups Romaine Hearts, shredded

3 tbsp Chimichurri Sauce

1 tbsp Apple Cider Vinegar

Preparation:

1. Combine everything except the steak and chimichurri in a bowl.

2. Serve with steak on the side and chimichurri for dipping.

3. Enjoy.

Dinner Recipes

The meal when the whole family gets together has to be yummy and highly enjoyable. See for yourself how even when trying to reverse a medical condition such as insulin resistance, you can enjoy a mouthwatering dinner.

Day 1: Lebanese Chicken Thighs

Ingredients:

4 Chicken Thighs

1 Onion, quartered

A handful of Baby Carrots

4 Garlic Cloves

Juice of 1 Lemon

2 Small Tomatoes, halved

Oregano, to taste

Black Pepper, to taste

Olive Oil

Preparation:

1. Heat your oven to 500 degrees F.

2. Place 2 tbsp olive oil in your cast-iron pan.

3. Place the chicken thighs; make sure to leave some space in between.

4. Place the carrots, onions, tomatoes and garlic in between.

5. Top with lemon juice and season.

6. Drizzle with olive oil.

7. Place in the oven and cook for 20 minutes.

8. Lower the heat to 350 degrees and cook for another 20 minutes.

9. Reduce the heat to 165 degrees and cook until the skin becomes crispy.

10. Enjoy.

Day 2: Sweet Pea Coconut Hash

Ingredients:

7 ounces Stringless Sugar Snap Pea Pods

4 tbsp Grass-Pastured Butter

1 tbsp Coconut Oil

1/8 tsp Cinnamon

1 tbsp Rosemary Oil

½ cup Shredded Coconut, unsweetened

Preparation:

1. Melt the butter in a pan over medium heat, and then add the coconut oil.

2. Chop the pea pods in 5 pieces.

3. Place the coconut in the pan.

4. Add rosemary oil and cinnamon.

5. Cook on low for about a minute.

6. Add the peas and mix well.

7. Cook them for 5 minutes over medium heat.

8. Enjoy.

Day 3: Tomato Shakshuka

Ingredients:

1 ½ pounds Cherry Tomatoes, halved

1 large Yellow Onion, chopped

1 Red Pepper, cut into thin strips

4 Organic Eggs

½ tbsp Cumin Seeds

2 fresh Thyme Sprigs

¼ cup Olive Oil

1 tbsp chopped Parsley

A pinch of cayenne Pepper

Preparation:

1. Preheat Your oven to 350 degrees F.

2. Place the tomatoes on a lined baking sheet.

3. Bake for half an hour until caramelized.

4. In a deep pan, dry roast the cumin seeds over medium heat.

5. Add the olive oil and sauté the onions on low.

6. Add the pepper along with the herbs.

7. Stir in the tomatoes.

8. Season with cayenne pepper.

9. When bubbly, break the eggs around the pan.

10. Cook on low for 10 minutes.

11. Serve and enjoy.

Day 4: Yellow Squash Pasta

Ingredients:

3 Summer Squash

¼ cup Fresh Parsley, chopped

Half a Lemon

1/3 cup chopped Almonds

2 tbsp Olive Oil

1tsp minced Garlic

Cayenne Pepper, to taste

Preparation:

1. Chop the ends off the squash.

2. With a vegetable peeler, peel long strips.

3. Heat the olive oil in a pan over medium heat.

4. Toss the squash into the pan.

5. Cook for 2 minutes, or until al dente.

6. Toss the parsley, almonds and garlic over.

7. Turn off the heat.

8. Squeeze the lemon.

9. Season with pepper.

10. Serve and enjoy.

Day 5: Pork Loin Stuffed with Spinach

Ingredients:

2 Pork Loin Cuts

1 cup of Fresh Spinach

1 tbsp Dijon Mustard

¼ cup Olive Oil

½ cup grated Parmesan Cheese

2 tsp minced Garlic

Garlic and HerbHavarti Cheese, to taste

Preferred Seasoning Mix, to taste

Preparation:

1. Preheat your oven to 400 degrees F.

2. In a Ziploc bag, place the Parmesan cheese, garlic, seasoning and olive oil.

3. Shake to combine.

4. Add the pork loin to the bag.

5. Shake to coat the pork loin well.

6. Place the pork loin on a lined baking dish.

7. Place the spinach on one-half of the pork loin.

8. Top the spinach with cheese.

9. Fold the pork loin with the other half.

10. Hold the meat closed with silicone baking bands.

11. Brush the meat with mustard.

12. Bake for about 45 minutes.

13. Enjoy.

Day 6: Cauliflower Crust Pizza

Ingredients:

2 cups grated (riced) Cauliflower

1 cup shredded Mozzarella Cheese

1 cup shredded Parmesan Cheese

1 tsp Garlic Powder

1 Egg, beaten

1 tsp Oregano

3 tbsp Tomato Paste

Preparation:

1. Preheat the oven to 450 degrees F.

2. Place the previously riced in a food processor cauliflower, in a microwave.

3. Microwave for 10 minutes.

4. Refrigerate the cauliflower until completely cooled.

5. Add the Parmesan cheese, half of the mozzarella cheese, the egg, and mix.

6. Add in the seasonings.

7. Pour the batter onto a baking sheet and flatten it with your hands.

8. Spread the tomato paste over.

9. Top with mozzarella cheese.

10. Bake for about 15-20 minutes.

11. Enjoy.

Day 7: Zucchini Aglio E Olio

Ingredients:

2 cups Zoodles (Zucchini Noodles)

3 tbsp Grass-Pastured Butter

¼ cup shaved Asiago Cheese

¼ cup grated Parmesan Cheese

1 tbsp minced Garlic

1 tbsp Olive Oil

1 tsp Red Pepper Flakes

1 tbsp chopped Red Pepper

1 tbsp chopped Basil

A Pinch of Cayenne Pepper

Preparation:

1. Melt the butter over medium heat in a skillet, then heat up the oil.

2. Add red pepper, the pepper flakes and garlic.

3. Add the zoodles and cook for 2 minutes.

4. Turn off the heat.

5. Add basil and Parmesan.

6. Transfer to a bowl.

7. Top with Asiago cheese.

8. Enjoy.

Healthy Habits for Vibrant Life

Eating the right kind of food will not help you achieve your goal if you overdo it. Know that at the beginning of this challenging journey you may frequently feel the pangs of hunger. It may occur because you will cut down on the calorie intake and abstain from certain types of food. Don't be fooled by the signals your tummy may send.

Here are some healthy habits that you can implement into your daily life to achieve your goal and live a healthy and vibrant life:

Always eat your breakfast within one hour of getting out of bed.

Your main meals should have 4-5 hours in between.

Never eat snacks before bedtime.

Never eat snacks on-the-go. Put them on a plate so you can have a pretty good picture of just how much you eat.

Always drink a glass of water before your meals.

Eat slowly. Don't rush while dining. Take your time, relax, take small bites and chew slowly.

Write down your meals. This will help you to keep track of your diet so you can easily spot if it lacks some type of food. Maybe you haven't been eating enough berries. Try to add them more into your diet.

Besides eating, here are some other tips that will contribute to improving your insulin sensitivity:

Do not forget to stay physically active. Even the best diet in the world will not have successful results if you stay inactive.

Avoid toxins. Yes, that also includes prescription drugs (unless you really need to take medications, of course). Try to approach your conditions as naturally as you can.

Expose yourself to sunlight regularly to optimize your vitamin D.

Reduce your stress as much as you can. Try some relaxation techniques whenever you have the time.

Conclusion

Learning is easy. You read a book, and you get to know things. Acting, on the other hand, is a completely different thing. It requires a strong will and motivation. Now that you have learned what you have to do in order to reverse your insulin resistance, please don't end your journey here.
Use this book as a pushing force that will guide you towards a much healthier life.

Finally, if you enjoyed this book, then I'd like to ask you for a favor, would you be kind enough to leave a review for this book on Amazon? It'd be greatly appreciated!

Thank you and good luck! ☺

www.ingramcontent.com/pod-product-compliance
Lightning Source LLC
Chambersburg PA
CBHW060218290526
45789CB00003B/1317